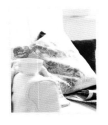

indulge

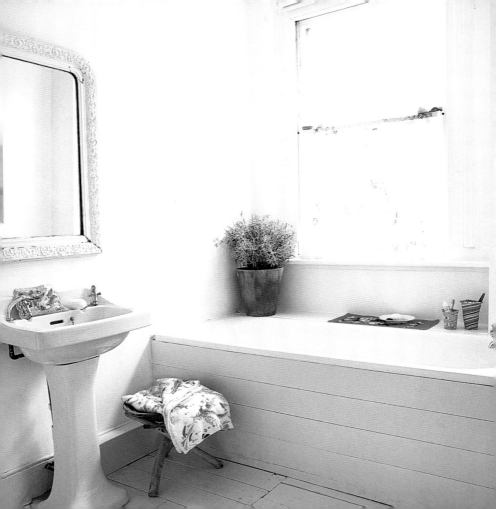

home spa
indulge

Liz Wilde

RYLAND
PETERS
& SMALL
LONDON NEW YORK

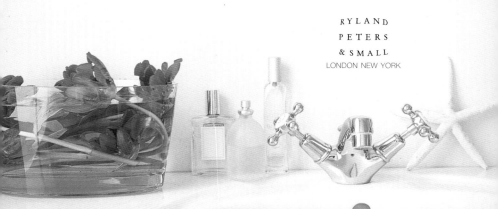

Designer Sarah Fraser
Senior Editor Clare Double
Picture Research Tracy Ogino
Production Paul Harding
Art Director Anne-Marie Bulat
Editorial Director Julia Charles

First published in the United States in 2006
by Ryland Peters & Small
519 Broadway, 5th Floor
New York, NY 10012
www.rylandpeters.com

ISBN-10: 1-84597-110-8
ISBN-13: 978-1-84597-110-6

If you are in any doubt about your health, please
consult your doctor before making any changes
to your usual dietary and wellbeing regime.
Essential oils are very powerful and potentially
toxic if used too liberally. Please follow the
guidelines and never use the oils neat on bare
skin, unless advised otherwise. This book is
not suitable for anyone during pregnancy.

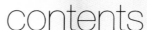

contents

introduction

When was the last time you spoiled yourself?

So many of us lead outwardly successful lives, yet we walk around feeling that life is tough and not much fun. We have "to do" lists that get no shorter, constant demands on our attention (cell phones make us contactable even when we're in the bath!), and a never-ending line of people wanting something from us. No wonder we end the day feeling tired and weary.

Are your evenings spent recovering for the next day? Do you spend your precious free time doing chores you don't enjoy, rather than on pleasures you do? A sure sign you've lost sight of the good life is when you ignore your best friend calling you up just so you can finish scrubbing the floor!

Indulging yourself is not selfish or vain. It's simply living your life the best you can, for as long as you can. And a life filled with pleasure is not just for women who can afford beauty treatments or spa weekends away. Everyone deserves to feel fabulous, and the good news is you can take care of your beauty, health, and wellbeing for a minimal cost.

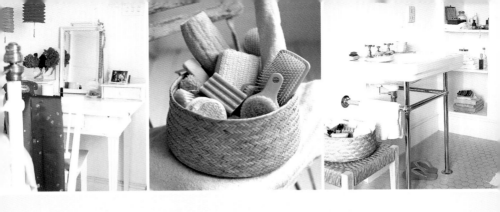

Looking good significantly boosts your self-esteem, and nothing destroys beauty faster than neglect. Luckily, recent research confirms what women have always known: that personal pampering is actually good for you. So indulging yourself every single day is now officially beneficial to your health!

This book will tell you how to include pleasure in your life even when you're carrying out the most mundane tasks. Show your body and mind how much you care, by making these indulgences part of your everyday life. And remember: by doing more of what makes you feel good, you'll also be looking after your health. Surely that's the only excuse you need?

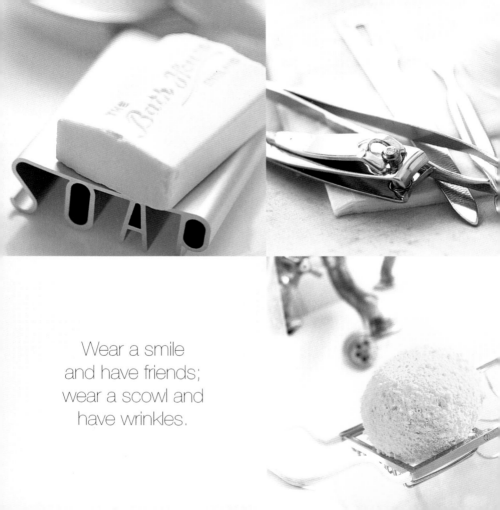

Wear a smile
and have friends;
wear a scowl and
have wrinkles.

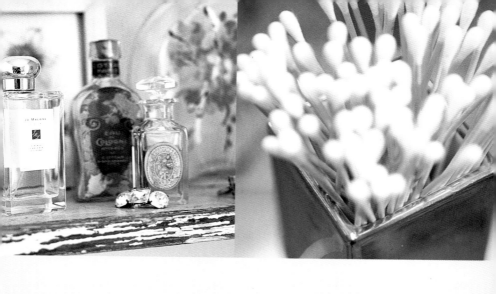

your looks

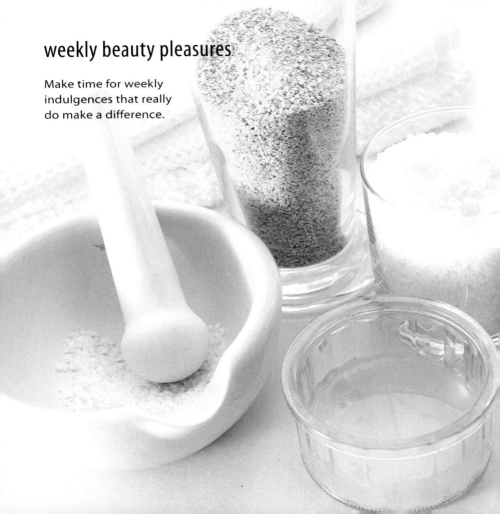

weekly beauty pleasures

Make time for weekly
indulgences that really
do make a difference.

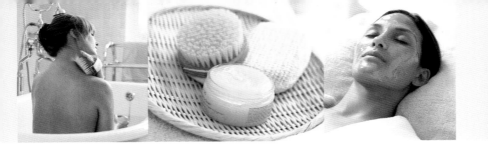

- **EXFOLIATION** guarantees brighter skin, as it removes dull, dead cells from the surface. Add a little salt, sugar, or oatmeal to your cleanser, and stroke rather than scour your damp skin for up to a minute before rinsing.

- **STEAMING** plumps up dry, dehydrated skin cells and softens blackheads. Pour boiling water over the juice of half a lemon, wait five minutes to cool, and then lean over it for no longer than three minutes.

- **MASKS** either deep-cleanse (choose clay-based masks for blocked pores) or moisturize (non-drying formulas will soften signs of aging). Apply to clean skin and leave on for the recommended time.

reasons to choose 100% natural

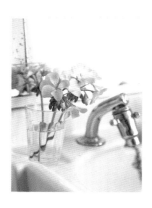

Treat your skin by choosing natural beauty products. What's all the fuss about? The chemicals used in many shampoos, conditioners, body lotions, and deodorants can also be found in antifreeze and brake fluid! And the foaming ingredient in many body gels, bubble baths, and facial washes is also responsible for the suds in engine degreasers, car-wash detergents, and floor cleaners. Up to 60% of chemicals applied to the skin are absorbed into the bloodstream, so it pays to be choosy about what's on your bathroom shelf. Look out for ranges that promise 100% natural and organic ingredients—they'll smell gorgeous, too.

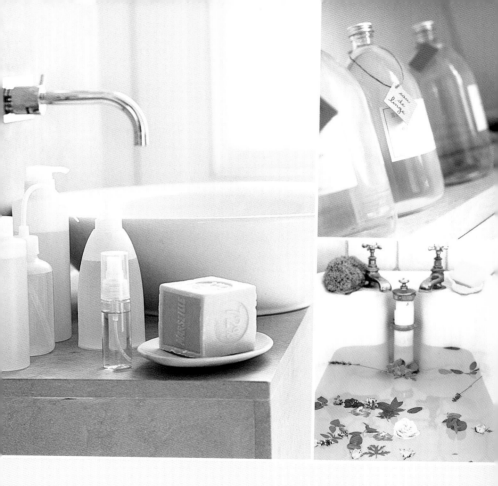

luxuries for low-morale days

Mix up your own luxury recipes. For a super-rich conditioning treatment courtesy of hair expert Philip Kingsley, add to your blender one large egg, two tablespoons of virgin olive oil, half a ripe avocado, a 2-ounce can of lumpfish roe (no need for caviar!) and a $\frac{1}{4}$ cup of heavy cream. Blend and apply to damp hair in sections, adding any leftovers to the ends. Cover your head in an old shower cap and leave for 15 minutes, or sleep in the mixture and wash it off in the morning. Heavy cream can also be used as a rich facial moisturizer as it's packed with vitamins A, D, and E. Or add two teaspoons of fine oatmeal to two teaspoons of heavy cream and you've got yourself a luxurious facial scrub that suits even sensitive skin.

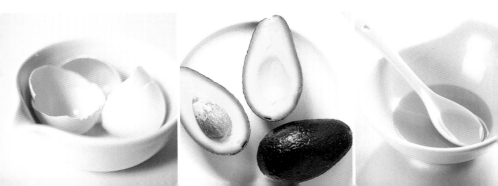

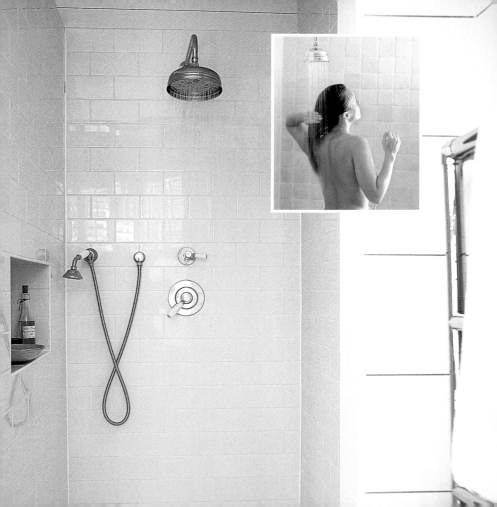

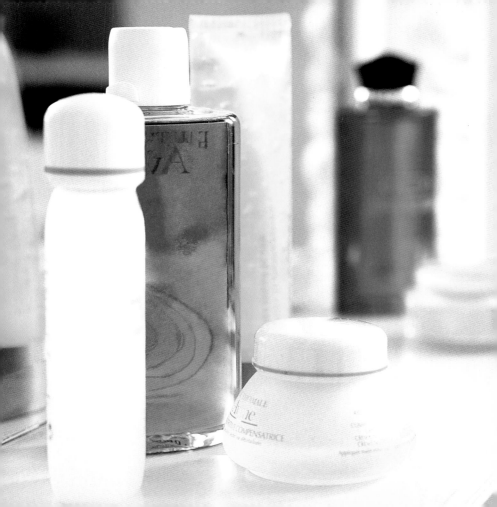

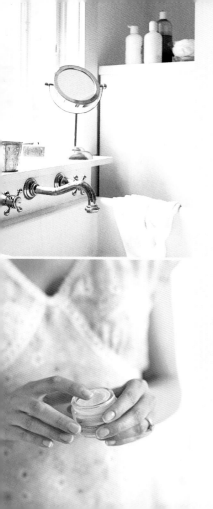

super skincare

Do believe (some) of the hype.
Super skincare ingredients such as
antioxidant vitamins A, C, and E (anti-
aging protectors), and AHAs (natural
exfoliators) really can improve the skin
you're in. Whether you choose a cream
or serum (one of the most effective
ways to penetrate your skin), this high
technology comes at a price. So if your
skin is sensitive, ask for a sample to try.
Or give yourself a patch test from the
in-store sample and check for irritation
(redness or itching) 24 hours later,
before investing your money.

overnight beauty treats

Simple overnight beauty treats can ensure
a more beautiful start to your day.

- Add **SHINE TO DULL HAIR** with an oil treatment.
  Warm two tablespoons of olive oil in a
  saucer above a small pan of boiling water
  and massage into your hair. Cover with
  a light shower cap (like the ones you get
  free in hotel rooms) and wash off in the
  morning by pouring shampoo directly
  onto your hair before rinsing. Shampoo
  a second time and condition.

- Break open a **VITAMIN E CAPSULE** and smear
  the oil over your lips for an overnight
  moisturizing mask. Any left over will
  condition dry cuticles, too.

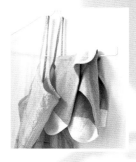

• Smother your feet in a rich moisturizer (petroleum jelly will do) and pop on a pair of old cotton socks to wear in bed. The heat generated during the night will ensure every last drop of moisture is absorbed by your skin for **SUPER-SMOOTH FEET** by morning. You can also give your hands an intensive moisture boost by applying your moisturizer and then wearing cotton gloves (available from drug stores) overnight.

• Skin experts are divided between recommending a rich cream or going naked (face-wise!) overnight so your skin can "rebalance" itself. If you have dry skin, then more moisture at night can only be a good thing, but if your skin's been stressed lately, **GIVE IT A BREAK** and it just might sort itself out.

put on a new face: fun in the department store

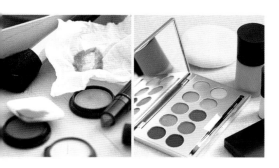

It's not just A-list celebrities who can get their make-up done by a professional.

Pop down to a department store beauty hall and let a make-up artist **CREATE A NEW FACE** for you. Gone are the days of the over-made-up assistant. Now premium brands employ professionals, ready to rescue a low-morale day. Watch and learn, then splash out on a key product and save the price of your lesson (the fee is redeemable against purchases). Most will give you a smudge sheet showing the colors used, so you can buy budget brands and copy the look for less.

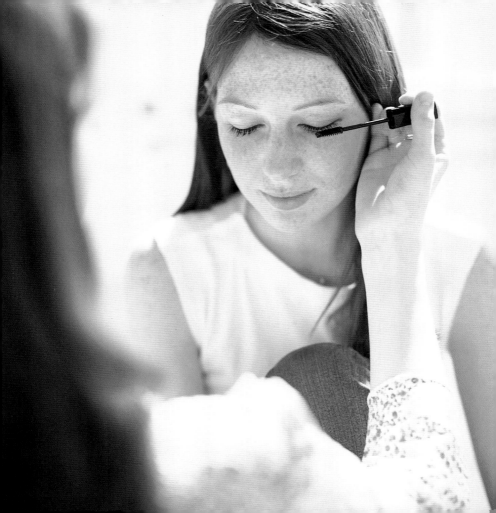

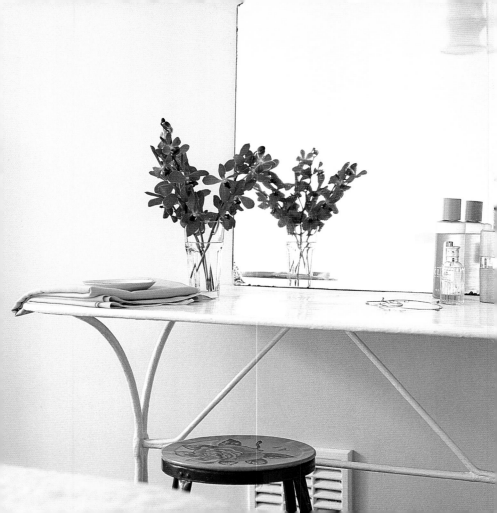

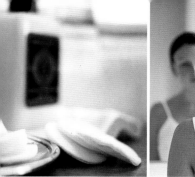
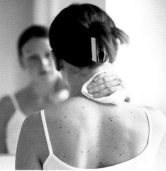
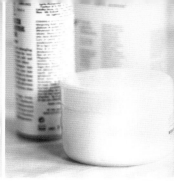

spoil-your-skin facial

For a spoil-your-skin cleanse, swap your usual cleanser for a pomade or balm. These natural oil formulas melt on contact with your skin and are removed with a wet washcloth or damp cotton pads. Skin experts say cleansing is the most important step in skincare, so don't skimp. Massage up from your collarbone using the pads of your fingers and medium-firm pressure (this will also boost circulation and bring tired skin back to life). Massage along your jawline to release tension that can cause headaches, and really work it into the grooves of your nose and chin. Allow the oil a minute to absorb every trace of dirt and make-up, and then remove gently for the softest skin you've ever had.

six quick fixes for less indulgent days

1 Have a mini water atomizer handy to spray your face throughout the day. A squirt before your morning moisturizer helps skin absorb more, a spray over make-up seals it all day, and a noontime squirt freshens make-up, softens fine lines, and wakes up a tired face.

2 Firming body creams work by intensively hydrating skin cells while gently exfoliating, both of which improve skin texture. Expect to see firmer, younger-looking skin in a matter of weeks, no diet required.

3 If you skip any skincare, make it toner (a splash of cool water will do). But for fast indulgence, you can't beat rosewater. It calms red, irritated skin and rehydrates all skin types, plus it smells gorgeous.

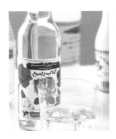

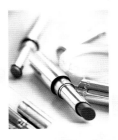

4   When you don't have time for make-up, red lipstick will bring your face to life. It's also a great color for diverting attention, so if your eyes are tired or your skin is blotchy, no one will notice!

5   On weary mornings when there's no time for cucumber slices, soak an absorbent cotton pad with cold milk and wipe it over lids to make eyes look whiter and brighter.

6   Every time you use hand cream, give yourself a mini hand massage. Rub the cream all over your hands using small circular movements and then gently pull your fingers to ease each joint.

your body

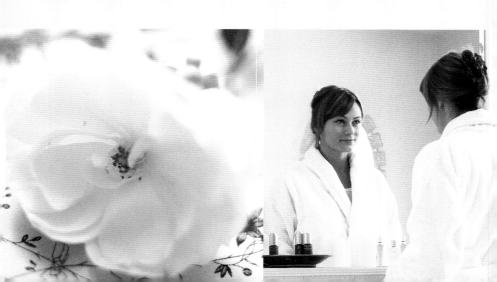

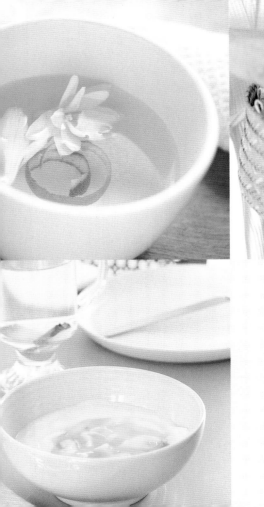
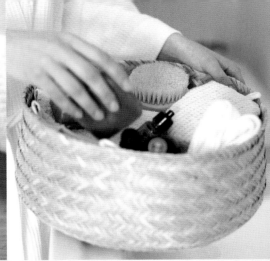

Happiness is
not being pained
in body nor
troubled in mind.
Thomas Jefferson

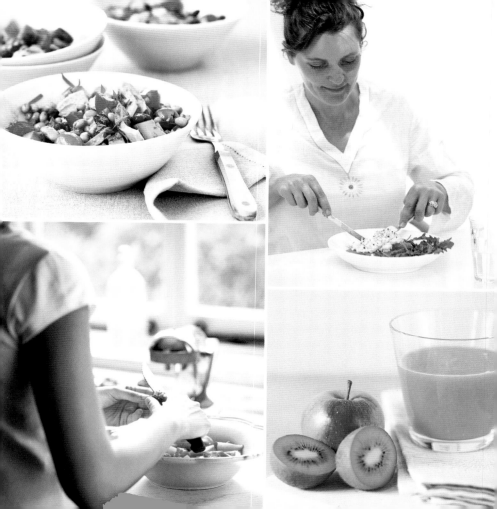

intuitive eating: improve your mood with food

There are thousands of books on what you should eat, but a far better idea is listening to your body. It's simple. Some foods increase your sense of wellbeing, while others leave you lethargic. Just eat any food you like and then notice how your body feels 45 minutes to an hour afterwards. If you're full of energy, you ate a food your body loves. If you're sleepy or sluggish, you ate a food your body's still working hard to digest. Once you see that food really is a mood-altering substance, you can

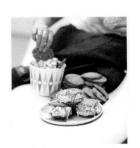

start to eat for how you want to feel. Ask yourself: how do I want to be in an hour's time? If the answer's "energetic," then choose food you know will take you there. If, on the other hand, you're planning an evening on the sofa, then maybe it's time to get the ice cream out…

happy hand massage

Indulge in a happy hand (and mind) massage. According to Taoists, pressure points on each finger correspond to specific emotions.

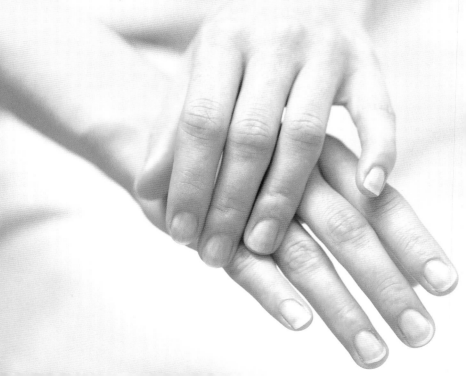

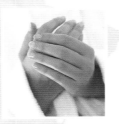

- **THUMB** = worry
- **INDEX FINGER** = sadness
- **MIDDLE FINGER** = impatience
- **RING FINGER** = anger
- **LITTLE FINGER** = fear

When you feel any of these emotions, massaging the relevant finger will give you **INSTANT RELIEF**. Begin by rubbing your hands together to generate warmth, then, using your right hand, wrap your fingers around the relevant finger on the left hand and start to massage it with your thumb. Concentrate on the sides and top just below the nail, taking as much time as you like, before repeating on the other hand.

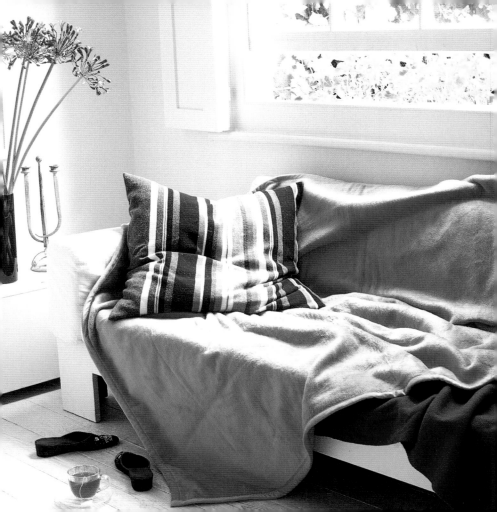

take a deep breath

Treat your body to a breathing mini-break.
Simply sit in a comfortable position, place
your hands on your knees and lower your chin
slightly. Inhale deeply through your
nose and then exhale quickly and
forcefully through your nose. Repeat
ten times, concentrating on the out-
breath so your inhale happens almost
without thinking. How does this help?
The forceful out-breath clears your
nasal passages and respiratory
system while calming a muddled
mind. Breathing this way also brings
huge supplies of oxygen into your
body, drawing out the same amount of carbon
dioxide, so you're left with cleaner blood. Add to
that a boost to your circulation, and you can see
why your body loves to deep-breathe.

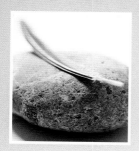

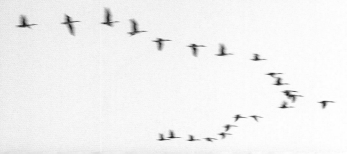

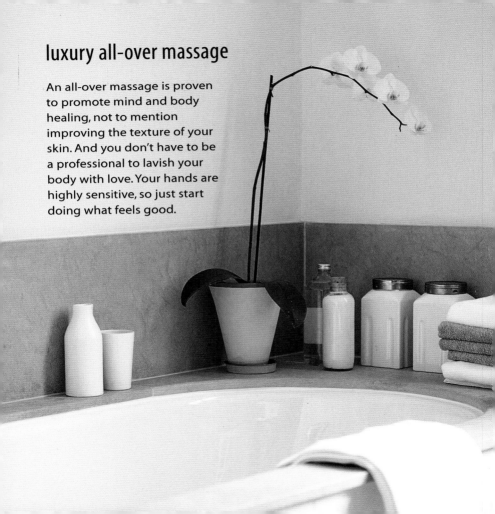

luxury all-over massage

An all-over massage is proven to promote mind and body healing, not to mention improving the texture of your skin. And you don't have to be a professional to lavish your body with love. Your hands are highly sensitive, so just start doing what feels good.

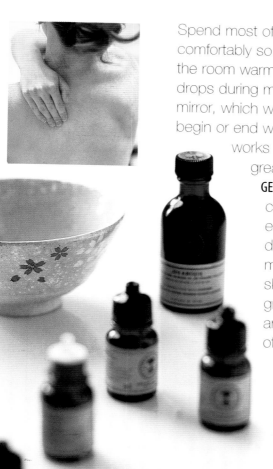

Spend most of the massage sitting comfortably so you can relax, and keep the room warm, as body temperature drops during massage. Avoid using a mirror, which will be distracting, and either begin or end with a warm bath. **STROKING** works well for relaxing, **KNEADING** is great for aching muscles, and **GENTLE PINCHING** is perfect for cellulite-prone areas as it encourages lymphatic drainage. Make your own massage blend for slippery skin with one tablespoon of grapeseed or soybean oil and no more than five drops of your favorite essential oil.

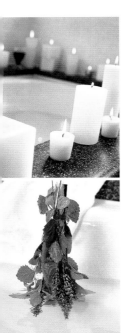

blissful bedtime

Night-time bathing guarantees a blissful bedtime, and may be the only time in the day when you get to be alone. Immersing yourself in warm water untightens tense muscles and makes you feel calmer and lighter, as it lowers blood pressure. Set the scene with whatever relaxes you—candles, music—and put a big towel over the warm radiator ready for when you step out. Add up to 10 drops of essential oil to the water (six if your skin's sensitive) and maximize the benefits by staying immersed for 20 minutes. Put a bath pillow or rolled-up towel behind your head so you can lie back comfortably, and inhale deeply (lavender or chamomile oils will make you sleepy). Once dry, spoil your skin with a rich body cream. For sensitive skin sufferers, this is the time to experiment with more adventurous products, as the skin on your body is usually far less reactive than your face. Then wrap yourself in a robe and head straight to bed—no jobs allowed.

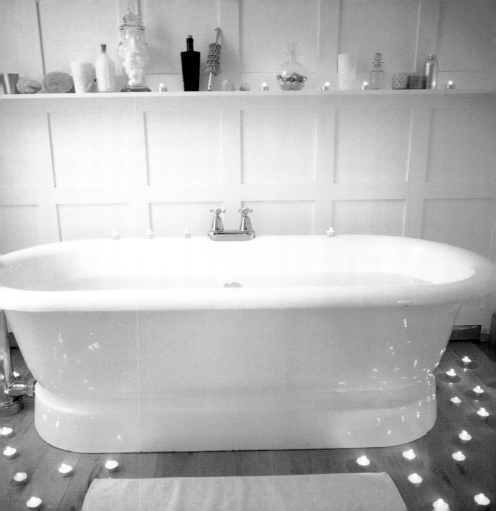

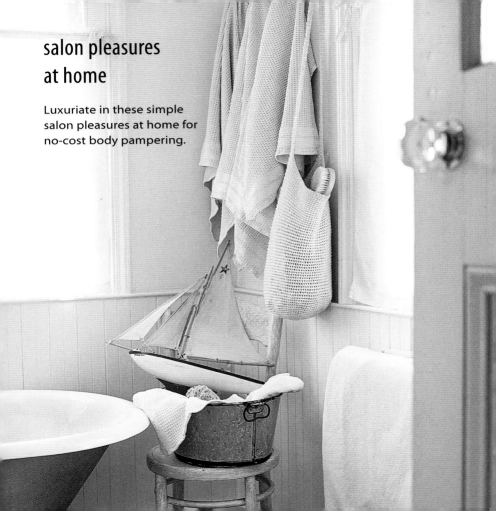

salon pleasures
at home

Luxuriate in these simple
salon pleasures at home for
no-cost body pampering.

- **SALT SCRUBS** literally lift off dry skin to expose the smooth layer underneath. Make your own with equal measures of sea salt and grapeseed or soybean oil (make the mixture smell nice with three drops of your favorite essential oil). Stand in the tub and massage all over, then either take a warm bath to prolong the detox benefits or shower off.

- Maximize any moisturizer by treating yourself to a **BODY WRAP** right afterwards. Warm a terrycloth bathrobe, plus socks and a towel, on the radiator. Then, after massaging in your oil or cream, slip on the robe and socks, place the towel over your lap, and relax in a chair for 20 minutes or until your cocoon has cooled.

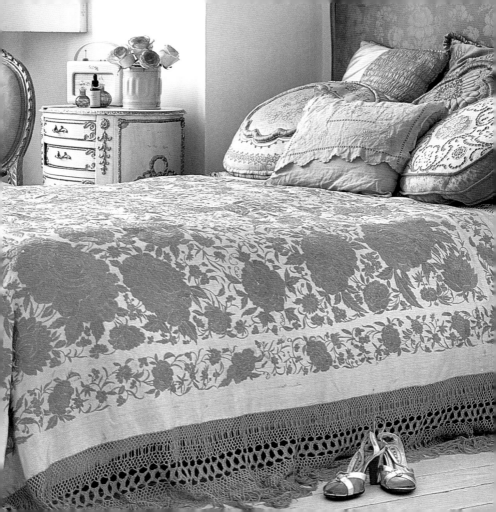

soothing scalp massage

A scalp massage soothes away tension any time, anywhere. Do it at night with oils and you'll also nourish your hair and scalp. The technique is simple. Using the balls of your fingers, start gently moving your scalp while keeping your fingers stationary (the less your scalp moves, the tenser it is). Slowly work around your head, continuing to move the scalp without moving your fingers (as your scalp becomes more relaxed, you can use more

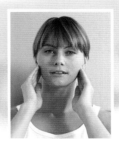

pressure). The base of your skull is worth special attention. Lean back onto your fingers and make small circles from the base of your skull out along your hairline and up and down both sides of your neck. If you're using oil (two tablespoons of any vegetable oil will do), leave it on for at least an hour or—even better—overnight.

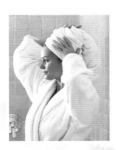

six ways to love your body

1   Be kind to your body by giving it what it was
    designed to eat. The enzymes in raw food are
    not only digested easily, but their calories are
    burned so efficiently it's almost impossible to
    get fat eating them! If nothing else, always eat
    something raw at the start of each meal.

2   Reducing your intake of sugary snacks and
    alcohol is hard to do (especially if you see no
    immediate benefit), but what better way is there
    to show you love your body than by taking very
    good care of it?

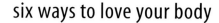

3 Show you love your skin (all twenty-one square feet of it) by eating what it loves: good-quality protein (eggs, fish, meat, tofu), lots of fresh vegetables and non-sugary fruits, and plenty of essential fatty acids (avocado, nuts, seeds, and oily fish). In just one week you'll reap the rewards.

4 Get plenty of *safe* sun exposure to boost your vitamin D levels, improve your immunity to infections, and boost serotonin, your brain's happy hormone.

5 Virtually any chemical that comes into contact with your skin can be absorbed, so reduce your exposure. Avoid processed foods (they're processed with chemicals) and artificial food additives such as MSG and sweeteners.

6 Calm your stress hormone cortisol (so destructive it's been called the death hormone!) by cutting down on coffee, getting plenty of exercise, and practicing daily deep breathing.

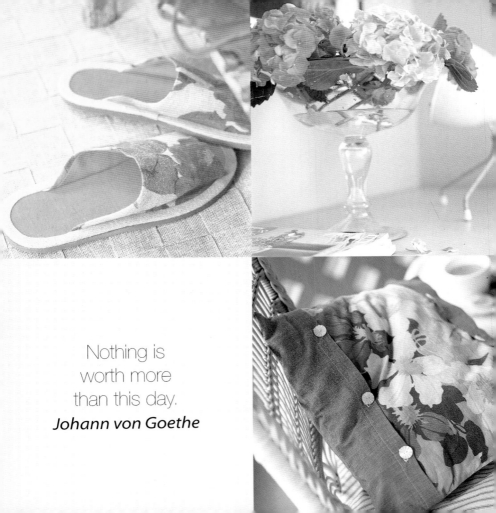

Nothing is
worth more
than this day.
Johann von Goethe

your life

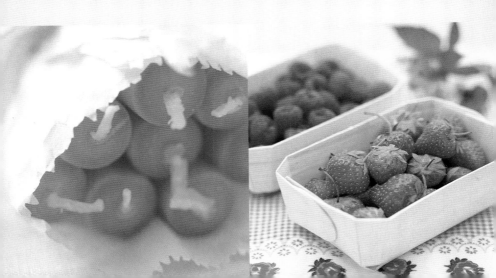

pamper your home

Pamper your home by making it smell delicious, but beware of synthetic products, which won't provide any therapeutic effect and may cause an allergic reaction.

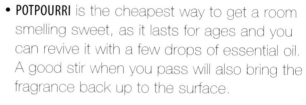

- **POTPOURRI** is the cheapest way to get a room smelling sweet, as it lasts for ages and you can revive it with a few drops of essential oil. A good stir when you pass will also bring the fragrance back up to the surface.

- **DIFFUSERS** (burners and lightbulb rings) vaporize essential oils into the air. The effect is subtle, but don't keep adding oil or you'll overdo it.

- **SPRAYS** made of essential oils are light and evaporate quickly, so shouldn't stain pillows or fabric, but test first on a dishcloth in case yours contain synthetic ingredients.

- **CANDLES** not only smell nice, they also make a room relaxing—and lighting them feels so indulgent. Buy good-quality candles made with pure essential oils and help them last longer by freezing before use. You need to let a candle burn at least one or two hours the first time, to give the oils a chance to be released. Keep the wick trimmed to a quarter of an inch for a cleaner burn.

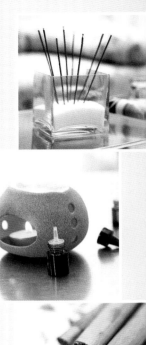

- **INCENSE** can contain synthetic perfume and even lighter fluid, so look for natural, botanical products. It can also be very potent and smoky, so save your sticks for summer, and if the smell overpowers (most are quite long), you can always open a window.

- **WHAT SMELL** to go where? For cozy, warm rooms (and winter), choose spices like orange, cinnamon, and sandalwood. Lighter rooms (and summer) suit florals like geranium or rose, and bedrooms love relaxing lavender.

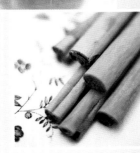

calm commuting

Whether your route to work involves sitting in traffic or being sandwiched on a train, recent research says that commuters can experience more stress than a fighter pilot going into battle. Stay calm by packing a de-stress essential oil like chamomile, lavender, or bergamot in your bag and sniffing it straight from the bottle, or take six drops of the Bach Flower Remedy impatiens on your tongue.

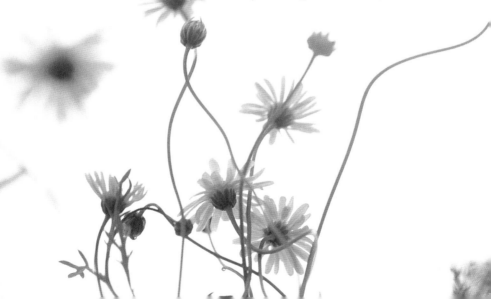

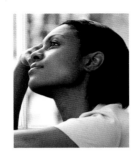

One way of lifting yourself out of the mayhem is to close your eyes and **VISUALIZE** yourself somewhere far more pleasurable. The trick is to imagine the scene in detail—how it looked, how it sounded, and especially how it felt. Breathe deeply as you relive the reality and chances are you'll start to relive those warm, fuzzy feelings, too. Stuck on a bus with no imagination or help in your bag? Press firmly on the **ACUPRESSURE POINT** between the two tendons on your inner arm, two to three finger-widths up from where your hand meets your wrist. Known as P6 on the pericardium meridian, it's the do-anywhere antidote to stress.

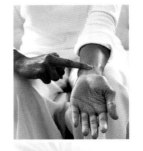

how to have a happy office

Your office needn't be a fun-free zone. Choose a scent you love but one you don't use at home, so it starts reminding you of work and creates positive vibes the

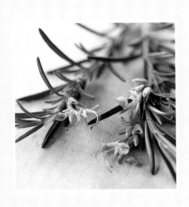

minute you step through the door. If your office smells good, everyone who visits will also feel good, which means you're far more likely to bring out the best in your colleagues as well. Choose light, fresh, citrus or spicy essential oils like peppermint (uplifting) or rosemary (great for concentration). But avoid anything relaxing—you don't want to be asleep by lunchtime. It's not only smell that can make nine to five a happier time. If you spend most of your day sitting at a desk, cheer it up with bright stationery (even if you have to buy it yourself) and a colored screensaver (or, better still, a vacation photo). No one enjoys looking at a gray desk all day.

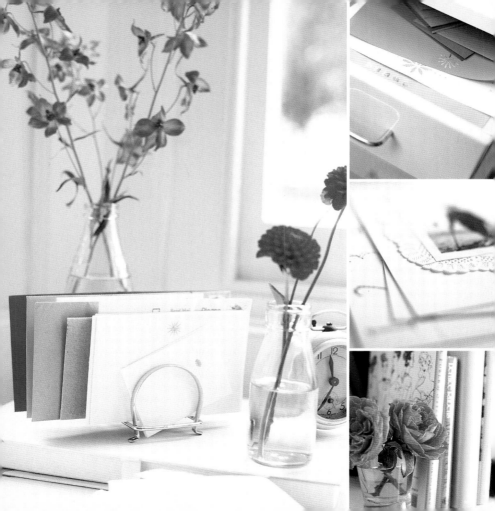

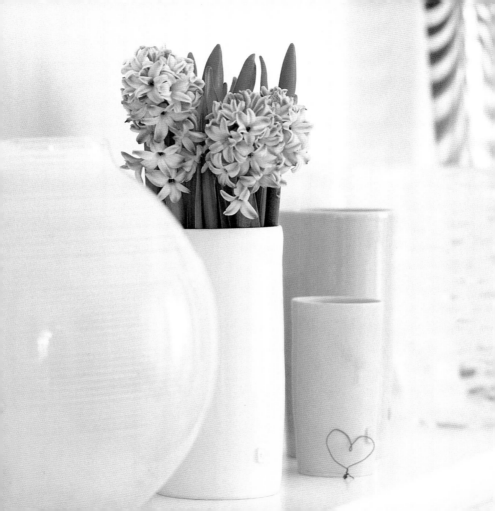

calorie-free ways to treat yourself

Not all pleasures are guilty. You just need to find other ways to treat yourself than overeating. In times of trouble we take refuge in bed, so sleep on top-quality bed linen (a cotton/linen mix is most luxurious) and change sheets once a week (it costs nothing). Plants aren't only healthy to have around the house (they absorb carbon dioxide from the air), but the right ones also smell wonderful. Choose freesias, hyacinths, lilies, or jasmine, or herbs like mint, lavender, basil, rosemary, or thyme (grow them in a cool area). And don't forget fun and laughter—they are life's shock absorbers, making us more resilient to everyday stresses and strains.

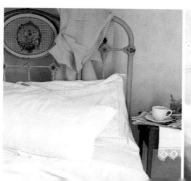
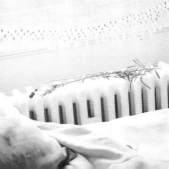

lunchtime lie-down

Afternoon siestas are the ultimate indulgence, but why save them for holidays when you can take a power nap at home, too?

Just two hours less sleep than the usual eight lowers your I.Q. by two points, but a 20-minute nap can **REBOOT YOUR BRAIN**, not to mention restore body and soul. Soothe yourself to sleep by consciously slowing your breathing, which is enough to put you into a light meditative state. Even if you don't drop off, this will still feel wonderfully relaxing.

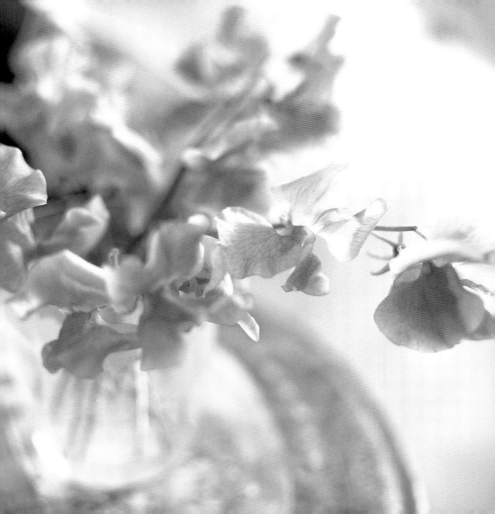

make everyday tasks indulgent treats

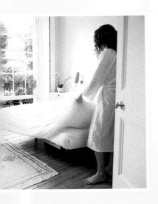

Domestic chores are very satisfying once they're done, so it's worth finding ways to make them more pleasurable.

- Play your favorite music as loudly as possible while you work. That way you'll hardly notice the dusting as you **DANCE** around the living room.

- Use essential oils rather than chemicals around your house. Mop floors and wipe surfaces with lemon- or lavender-scented water to add **FRAGRANCE** and neutralize microbes. Scent your sheets in the linen closet by sprinkling on a few drops of essential oil, or fill a spray bottle with water and add a few drops of lavender oil to squirt over your laundry as you iron.

- Use chores as a way to fill up time while a **BEAUTY TREATMENT** gets to work. Pile your hair high in a conditioning treatment and vacuum the house. Paint your toenails and iron your way through the week's laundry while you're waiting for the polish to dry. Smooth on fake tan, then dust in the nude while it sinks into your skin.

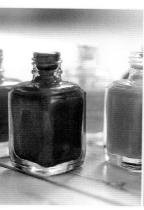
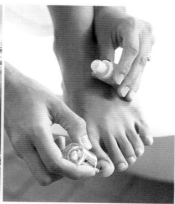
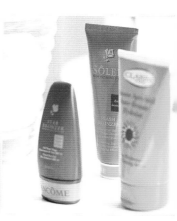

posh up your pampering

Clean up your beauty act by wiping around all your clogged-up bottles of lotions and potions. Throw away what you don't use, to make way for new purchases—a great excuse to treat yourself. A bathroom blitz not only results in time saved in the morning, but you'll also discover half-used and forgotten beauty buys collecting dust at the back of the drawer.

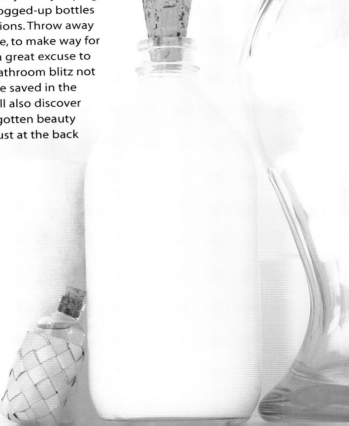

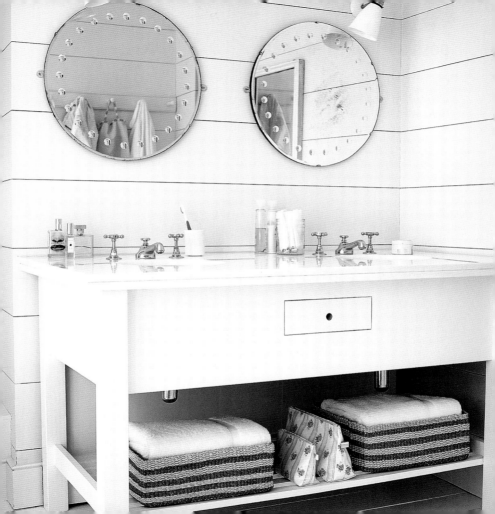

six habits to make each day a pleasure

1   Take very good care of yourself every single day.
    It's much easier to be positive about life when you're
    treating yourself well.

2   Physical contact with friends, loved ones, and even
    pets is an instant pick-me-up. Need proof? Waitresses
    get higher tips from customers if they touch them on
    the arm as they hand over the bill!

3   Everyone gets a good feeling from helping someone
    else, whether it's a work colleague who's stuck or a
    mother struggling up the stairs with a stroller. The more
    positive energy you put out, the more you'll get in return.

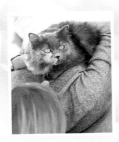

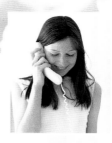

4   Talk to at least one good friend every day. Connection with friends is good for the soul, because it gives us a sense of belonging.

5   Ditch the rock music. A recent study found that adults who listened regularly to mood music felt less fatigue and depression after just six weeks, plus the effect lasted a full seven weeks afterwards.

6   Stress doesn't seem so bad when you remind yourself of the things that are right in life. Taking just 60 seconds a day to stop and appreciate the good stuff will make a huge difference to your mood.

useful addresses

Aveda
866 823 1425
for stores
www.aveda.com

Barneys New York
660 Madison Avenue
New York, NY 10021
212 826 8900
www.barneys.com

Bath & Body Works
800 395 1001 for stores
www.bathandbody
    works.com

Bloomingdale's
1000 Third Avenue
New York, NY 10022
212 705 2000
www.bloomingdales.com

Crabtree & Evelyn
800 272 2873 for stores
www.crabtree-evelyn.com

Crate & Barrel
650 Madison Avenue
New York, NY 10022
800 967 6696 for stores
www.crateandbarrel.com

Giorgio Armani Cosmetics
www.giorgioarmani.com

Laura Mercier Cosmetics
www.lauramercier.com

**National Women's Health
Resource Center**
157 Broad Street, Suite 315
Red Bank, NJ 07701
877 986 9472
www.healthywomen.org
Information resource
helping women to pursue
healthy lifestyles.

Origins
www.origins.com

**Oshadhi natural and
organic aromatherapy**
+44 1223 242242
www.oshadhi.co.uk

**Philip Kingsley's
Trichological Clinic**
54 Green Street
London W1
+44 20 7629 7629

Sephora
2103 Broadway
New York, NY 10023
212 362 1500
www.sephora.com

credits

Key: ph=photographer, a=above, b=below, r=right, l=left, c=center

Endpapers & 1 ph Polly Wreford; 2 ph Debi Treloar; 3–4 ph Polly Wreford; 5 ph Debi Treloar; 7l ph Polly Wreford; 7c & r ph Dan Duchars; 8al ph Andrew Wood; 8ar & b ph David Montgomery; 9l ph Claire Richardson; 9r ph Andrew Wood; 10 ph David Montgomery; 11l & r ph Daniel Farmer; 11c ph Dan Duchars; 12 ph Polly Wreford; 13l & br ph Caroline Arber; 13ar ph Chris Everard; 14l ph Tara Fisher; 14c ph Daniel Farmer; 14r ph Peter Cassidy; 15 background ph Jan Baldwin; 15 inset & 16 ph Daniel Farmer; 17a ph Chris Tubbs / Maureen Kelly's house in the Catskills, New York; 17b & 18 ph Dan Duchars; 19 background ph David Montgomery; 19 inset & 20l ph James Merrell; 20r ph Daniel Farmer; 21 ph Dan Duchars; 22 ph Polly Wreford; 23l ph Chris Everard; 23c & r ph Dan Duchars; 24 inset & 24–25 background ph David Montgomery; 25 inset ph Dan Duchars; 26l ph Claire Richardson; 26r ph Daniel Farmer; 27al & b ph David Montgomery; 27ar ph Dan Duchars; 28al ph Nicki Dowey; 28ar & bl ph Dan Duchars; 28br ph Noel Murphy; 29 ph Debi Treloar; 30 ph Dan Duchars; 31 ph Polly Wreford; 32 ph David Montgomery; 33 background ph Chris Tubbs; 33 inset ph Jan Baldwin; 34 ph Caroline Arber / Rosanna Dickinson's home in London; 35 ph Dan Duchars; 36–37 ph David Montgomery; 38 ph James Merrell; 39 ph Dan Duchars; 40 ph Daniel Farmer; 41 background ph David Montgomery; 41 insets ph Daniel Farmer; 42 ph Peter Cassidy; 43 ph Nicki Dowey; 44a ph Polly Wreford; 44b ph James Merrell; 45l ph David Brittain; 45r ph Noel Murphy; 46 background ph William Lingwood; 46 inset & 47b ph Claire Richardson; 47a ph Dan Duchars; 47c ph Daniel Farmer; 48–49 background ph David Montgomery; 49 insets ph Daniel Farmer; 50 ph Peter Cassidy; 51 ph Polly Wreford; 52 & 53r inset ph James Merrell; 53 background & l inset ph Polly Wreford / Linda Garman's home in London; 54 background ph Debi Treloar; 54 inset ph Daniel Farmer; 55 ph Polly Wreford; 56 background ph David Montgomery; 56 inset, 57l & r ph Dan Duchars; 57c ph Daniel Farmer; 58 ph David Montgomery; 59 ph Jan Baldwin / Sophie Eadie's family home in London; 60 background ph Debi Treloar; 60 inset ph James Merrell; 61 background ph Claire Richardson; 61 inset ph Dan Duchars; 62 ph David Montgomery; 63 ph James Merrell; 64 ph Tom Leighton.

acknowledgments

The author would like to thank all her
wonderful friends and family.

Visit Liz Wilde's website at
www.wildelifecoaching.com to subscribe
to her free Monthly Motivator Mail.

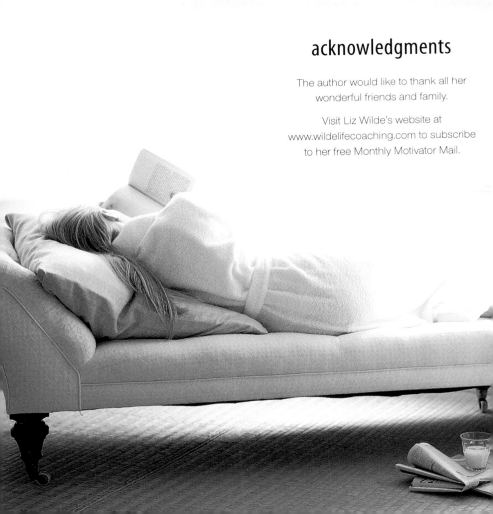